This notebook belongs to:

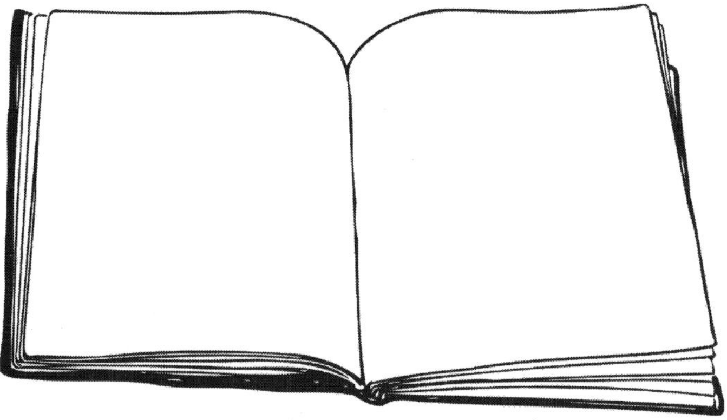

Made in the USA
Monee, IL
08 March 2022

92525651R00072